'Easy Yo[

*Your Ultimate Beginners Guide
to Understanding Yoga and
Leading a Disease-Free Life
through Routine Yoga Practice*

by

Advait

Disclaimer and FTC Notice

Easy Yoga: Your Ultimate Beginners Guide to Understanding Yoga and Leading a Disease-Free Life through Routine Yoga Practice
Copyright © 2015, Advait. All rights reserved.

ISBN-13: 978-1515003021

ISBN-10: 1515003027

medical problems without the advice of a physician, either directly or indirectly.

The intent of the author is only to offer information of a general nature to help you in your quest for emotional, spiritual and physical well being. In the event you use any of the information in this book for yourself, which is your constitutional right, the author and the publisher assume no responsibility for your actions.

Under no circumstances will any legal responsibility or blame be held against the publisher for any reparation, damages, or monetary loss due to the information herein, either directly or indirectly. The information herein is offered for informational purposes solely, and is universal as so. The presentation of the information is without contract or any type of guarantee assurance.

Adherence to all applicable laws and regulations, including international, federal, state, and local governing professional licensing, business practices, advertising, and all other aspects of doing business in the US, Canada, or any other jurisdiction is the sole responsibility of the purchaser or reader.

Neither the author nor the publisher assumes any responsibility or liability whatsoever on the behalf of the purchaser or reader of these materials.

Advait

Any perceived slight of any individual or organization is purely unintentional.

Easy Yoga

Contents

Advait

Easy Yoga

The True Meaning of Yoga

There is a common and popular belief that 'Yoga' is an Indian ritual which is all about performing difficult physical exercises for maintaining health and curing diseases.

This is a MYTH!!

Actually, Sound Health is a side-effect of Yoga.

Surprising!!! But true.

The word 'Yoga' literally means *to unite ourselves with our higher self* - an entirely meta-physical objective which can be achieved through a Discipline of Physical exercises (Asana's) coupled with Meditation exercises (*Dhyana*) and Breathing exercises (Pranayam). When we perform those exercises we get in shape and achieve good health.

Yoga is not something to be performed or practiced, it is to be achieved.

Yoga is the destination and the path to it is through a disciplined practice of physical exercises, meditation and breathing exercises.

Maharshi Patanjali, in his revolutionary work *'Paatanjal YogaSutra'* prescribes an eight-fold path to achieve Yoga, known as *Ashtang Yoga*.

['Paatanjal YogaSutra' is considered to be the most comprehensive book on Yoga and it forms the basis and reference of all the Yoga methodologies practiced throughout the world today.]

The Ashtang Yoga [eight-fold path to yoga], given by Maharshi Patanjali is as follows:

Yama

The moral virtues that one should possess as they are considered to be essential for one's initiation on the path to yoga.

Niyama

It involves being knowledgeable and aware about your surroundings and then studying your-self to form an essential discipline which you would adhere to.

Asana

Understanding and Performing the required physical exercises, this is the core of your yoga practice.

Pranayam

It is all about breath control, which enhances the life energy which governs the existence of a being and balances the mental energy.

Pratyahar

Sensory inhibitions which internalize the consciousness and prepare your mind to take action.

Dharana

It involves inculcating an extended mental focus to concentrate on only those things that are essential.

Dhyana

It involves meditation, paying attention to your breathing and thus focusing only on yourself.

Samadhi

Becoming one with the object of your contemplation and experiencing spiritual liberation.

Advait

Yama and Niyama are essential for inculcating the needed discipline and establish a strict routine.

Asana is the crucial physical part, which subjects your body to essential physical movements through different exercises.

Pranayam and Pratyahar are needed to guide us through the various breathing exercises and for making us aware of the internal spiritual changes as we ascend along the path to Yoga.

Dharana and Dhyana stages prepare us mentally and spiritually to concentrate inwards by using various meditation exercises.

Samadhi is the culmination stage where one achieves Yoga.

A Brief History of Yoga

Before going any further let's look back at where it all began.

To tell you the truth…. No one knows!!

The foundation of Yoga as a science is attributed to *Maharshi Patanjali* who lived in India in 3rd Century B.C.

But, archeological excavations in the Indus Valley civilization sites have unearthed sculptures and idols depicting various Asana's (physical exercise positions) suggested in Yoga and these idols date back to around 3000 years B.C.

Also, information about various aspects of Yoga can be found in Vedic texts like; Shwetashwatrupanishad,

Chaandogyopanishad,

Kaushitki Upanishad,

Maitri Upanishad etc.

This information was scattered all over and Maharshi Patanjali, compiled these nuggets into a streamlined and strict science of Yoga or should I say he compiled this scattered information into a way of life called *Yoga* through his work 'Paatanjal YogaSutra'

After Maharshi Patanjali,

Maharshi Swatwaram wrote 'Hatapradipika' (meaning - One Which Illuminates the Path of Hatha Yoga , i.e. the physical aspect of Yoga) in the 13th Century A.D.

And, Maharshi Gherand wrote 'Gherandsanhita' around the same time.

Almost all the Yoga methodologies practiced world-over today regard Maharshi Patanjali's work as their reference.

Importance of a *Yoga Routine*

I like to keep all my books absolutely fluff free and concise. I promise you, this book will be no different.

I will not waste 10 pages in convincing you about how amazing Yoga is and how you can benefit from practicing it. But, I will tell you this...

*If you want to live at least a **100 years of disease-free life** and want the same for your loved ones, the only thing that can guarantee it is a Yoga Routine.*

Many western scholars claim that Ancient Indian Seer's (Maharshi's) had a life span of well over a century and they attribute this longevity to a regular practice of Yoga by these Maharshi's.

For e.g.: Maharshi Vyaas, is attributed to compiling and categorizing the scattered Vedic Knowledge and Wisdom into the four Veda's (that's the reason why is also called as Maharshi Ved Vyaas), he is also attributed for writing 'Mahabharata' (mind you, the 'Bhagavad Gita' is but a small part of Mahabharata) and numerous other works, and many scholars and historians have concluded that it is not possible to do all this in an average life span of 60-70 years, so he had to have lived well over a century.

Such similar comparisons can also be drawn true to numerous other Philosophers, Thinkers and Acharya's of Vedic India.

The bottom-line is, a well established, sincere and disciplined *Yoga Routine* is the best medical insurance you can have for yourself and your family.

Types of Yoga Exercises

It is impossible to make a general classification of Yoga Asana's (exercises), as each Asana can be classified into multiple sub-categories, for e.g.;

A. Asana's can be classified depending upon whether you hold your breath in while performing the exercise, you exhale and perform the exercise or you maintain your normal rate of breathing.

B. Asana's can be classified depending upon whether you perform it standing, sitting or lying down on the mat.

C. Asana's can also be classified depending upon the parts of the body being extended and stretched.

For our ease and understanding, in this book and in the subsequent 'Yoga Routine' series, we broadly classify Asana's into Three (3) categories:

I. Dhyanasana's:

Asana's which don't involve much physical movement, but focus more on mental focus and concentration, with a hint of meditation, viz. *Swastikasan.*

II. Vyayamasana's: (vyayam = physical exercise)

Asana's which mainly focus on physical movements and stretching, viz. *Taulasan.*

III. Vishrantiasana's: (Vishranti = Rest/Relaxation)

Asana's which are used to relax and rest your body after performing physical Asana's, viz. *Shavasan.*

Some Essential Precautions

Here are some precautions and rules you need to follow if you wish to achieve best results;

1. Yoga is very helpful if done in the Morning and on an empty stomach (don't eat anything, you can drink water). If you cannot make time in the morning, you can practice it in the evening but make sure that you practice it after 4 to 4 ½ Hrs. of having your meals.

2. When you get up in the morning , have a glass of water, visit the toilet (what I mean is, take a poop), take a shower and then do Yoga, as water will rejuvenate your system and taking a shower will warm up your body for the exercises you are about to perform.

3. Understand this; You are the only essential for Yoga and not your clothes. I find all the recent 'yoga attire' fad to be pointless. All you need is a simple mat to sit on, A Pajama and a loose T-shirt which don't restrict your movements while you perform the Asana's.

4. Take your time while performing the Asana's, don't hurry through the exercises as if you are on a deadline. Remember, 'Yoga is for You...You are not for Yoga'. If you find yourself short on time,

don't perform all the listed exercises in a hurry, practice only a few that you can in that short time, but slowly and steadily.

5. Don't let your mind wander off while doing the Asana's, concentrate on your movements instead. A very easy trick is to concentrate on your breathing.

6. Women should not perform Yoga during menstruation.

7. A pregnant woman should not practice the Asana's from the 4th Month of her pregnancy.

8. Avoid performing Asana's back to back in quick succession, rest for at least 5-6 seconds between two Asana's.

9. After your Yoga session, do not eat or drink anything for at least 25 to 30 min.

10. If you have had a bone broken in the past and now its mended, still, don't submit that appendage to too much strain while performing an Asana.

11. Commit to routine practice of Yoga, make it a way of life.

Warm-up Exercises before you Begin

Like any other exercise, warming up before performing Yoga exercises (Asana's) is very important as it conditions your body to get used to the physical movements and stretching movements without bruising or hurting a muscle.

Look at the warm-up as an essential catalyst which enables your body to extract the full benefits of an Asana.

Warm-Up Exercise #1

Heel Raise:

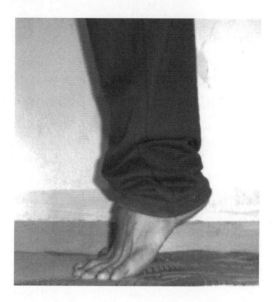

Stand straight/erect, without slouching.

Your feet should be close together.

Raise your body up on your toes (you can support yourself by holding on to a support).

Hold the position for 4-5 seconds and then slowly return to your original standing position.

Repeat it 7-8 times.

Easy Yoga

Warm-Up Exercise #2

Reverse Arch:

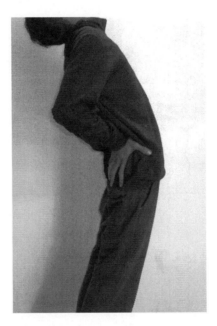

Stand straight/erect, without slouching.

Your feet should be around 1 foot apart.

Keep both your hands on your hips with your fingers pointing downwards.

Bend backwards at the waist, supporting your lower back with your hands.

(bend backwards as much as you can without hurting yourself)

Advait

Hold the position for 4-5 seconds and then slowly return to your original standing position.

Repeat it 5-6 times.

Warm-Up Exercise #3

Leg Raise:

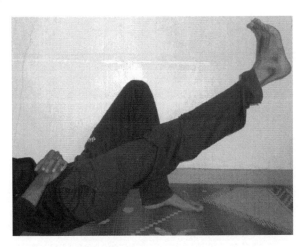

Lie on your back.

Keep one leg straight and the other bent at the knee.

Now slowly lift the straight leg up to a height of 10-12 inches from the ground and hold it there for 3-4 seconds.

Slowly take the raised leg down and repeat with the other leg.

This way, raise both the legs 7-8 times.

Warm-Up Exercise #4

Stretching Hamstring:

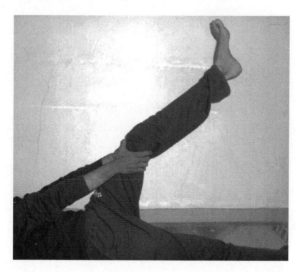

Lie on your back.

Keep one leg straight and the other bent at the knee.

Put your hands around the upper part of the bent leg. (refer image)

Slowly straighten the leg until you feel a stretch in the back of the upper leg and hold it for 3-4 seconds.

Slowly take the raised leg down and repeat with the other leg.

Easy Yoga

This way, raise both the legs 7-8 times.

Warm-Up Exercise #5

Single Knee Pull:

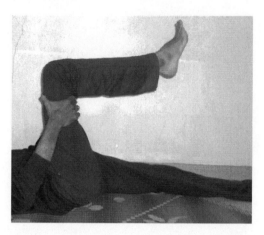

Lie on your back.

Keep one leg straight and the other bent at the knee.

Put your hands around the upper part of the bent leg. (refer image)

Now holding your thigh behind the knee, pull your knee up to your chest and hold for 3-4 seconds.

Slowly take the raised leg down and repeat with the other leg.

This way, raise both the legs 7-8 times.

Warm-Up Exercise #6

Double Knee Pull:

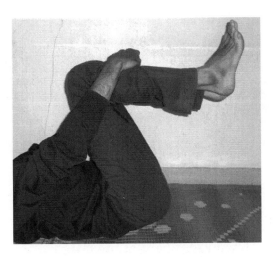

Lie on your back.

Keep both your legs bent at the knee.

Put your hands around the upper part of the bent legs. (refer image)

Now holding your thighs behind the knees, pull your knees up to your chest and hold for 3-4 seconds.

Slowly take the raised legs down.

Repeat for 7-8 times.

Warm-Up Exercise #7

Hip Roll:

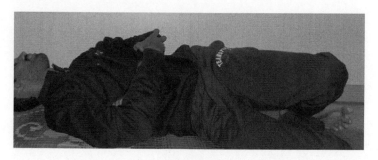

Lie on your back.

Keep both your legs bent at the knee.

Cross your arms over your chest.

Now, turn your head to the left while turning your knees to the right.

Invert and repeat.

10 Basic *Yoga Asana's* to get You started on the Path to Yoga

Yoga Asana #1

Swastikasan/Asana of Swastika

The Sanskrit word *Swastika* means pious. (do not confuse a swastika with the 'nazi symbol' which is an 'inverted' swastik)

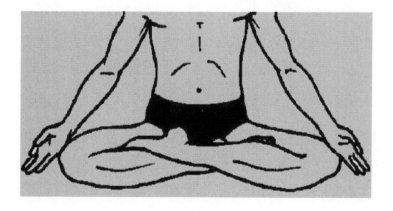

Method:

Sit comfortably on the mat.

Sit straight, with your spine erect. Do not slouch over.

Now fold your legs is such a way that the toes of your right foot are pressed between the thigh and calf muscle of the left leg and the toes of your left foot are pressed between the thigh and calf muscle of the right leg. (refer image)

Rest your hands on your knees, with your palms facing upwards.

Touch the tip of the index finger to the tip of the thumb on both your hands. (this hand gesture is called a 'Dnyanmudra')

Keep breathing slowly and comfortably while you perform this Asana.

Duration:

This Asana (position) should be held for 2-3 minutes.

Repeat at least 3 times for best results.

Uses:

-This Asana enhances mental strength

-It helps in calming down your mind.

-It strengthens your nervous system.

-On the physical front, This Asana helps in keeping Diabetes under control.

-It also strengthens the Pancreas.

Advait

Yoga Asana #2

Padmasan/ Asana of Lotus

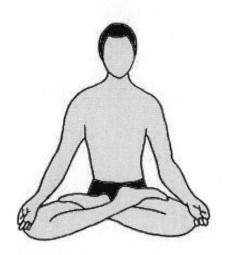

Method:

Sit comfortably on the mat with your legs stretched out front.

Now, fold your right leg and place the foot on your left thigh with the base of the right foot (palm of the foot) facing upwards. (refer the image)

Then, fold your left leg and place the foot on your right thigh with the base of the left foot (palm of the foot) facing upwards.

Easy Yoga

The heel of both your feet should be touching the base of the opposite thighs.

Rest your hands on your knees, with your palms facing upwards.

Touch the tip of the Index finger to the tip of the Thumb on both your hands.

Keep breathing slowly and comfortably while you perform this Asana.

(You will feel some pain when you are just starting out but with 4-5 days of regular practice, you should feel no discomfort.)

Duration:

When you perform this Asana for the first few days, do it only for 8-10 seconds at a stretch. But, with practice you'll fell more supple and flexible and then perform it for 1-2 minutes at a stretch.

Uses:

-It works miraculously well in treating Arthritis.

- It enhances your digestive capabilities.

- It cures any stomach aches you have and increase hunger.

Advait

-It strengthens your heart.

-It imparts flexibility to all the organs below the waistline.

-Regular practice of this Asana induces mental & spiritual calmness.

Yoga Asana #3

Taulasan/Asana of Scales

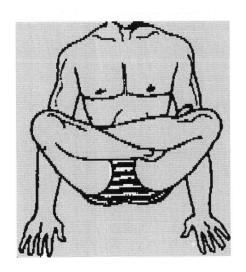

Method:

Sit comfortably on the mat with your legs stretched out front.

Now, fold your right leg and place the foot on your left thigh with the base of the right foot (palm of the foot) facing upwards. (refer the image)

Then, fold your left leg and place the foot on your right thigh with the base of the left foot (palm of the foot) facing upwards.

Advait

The heel of both your feet should be touching the base of the opposite thighs.

Keep both of your hands on the ground with your palms facing down.

Take a deep breath and don't exhale. (*Kumbhak*)

Now raise yourself up from the ground by putting all your weight on your hands. (refer image)

Hold this position for 3-4 seconds, then return to the normal position and exhale out slowly.

Duration:

This Asana takes 10-12 seconds to perform and you can repeat it 4-5 times.

Uses:

-This Asana strengthens your arms.

-It is very effective in curing back pain and shoulder pain.

-This is a very effective Asana for who those need to continuously type something sitting at their desk in their line of work. (writers, data -entry professionals etc.)

Yoga Asana #4

Parvatasan/Asana of Mountain

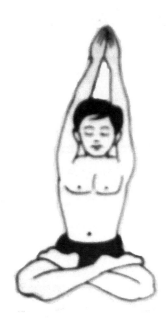

Method:

Sit comfortably on the mat with your legs stretched out front.

Now, fold your right leg and place the foot on your left thigh with the base of the right foot (palm of the foot) facing upwards. (refer the image)

Then, fold your left leg and place the foot on your right thigh with the base of the left foot (palm of the foot) facing upwards.

The heel of both your feet should be touching the base of the opposite thighs. (This is how you sit in *Padmasan*)

Now raise your hands up above your head and bring your palms together form a *Namaste* gesture (refer the image). [Namaste – Indian form of Salutation]

Extend your arms up, as much as you can without breaking the contact between your palms.

Take a deep breath, keep the air in for a few seconds and then exhale slowly. Bring your hands down and be in the original position.

All the while keep your body straight and aligned.

Duration:

This Asana takes 10-52 seconds to perform and you can repeat it 5-6 times.

Uses:

-This Asana strengthens the Muscles of your chest, abdomen and upper back.

Easy Yoga

-It is very helpful in strengthening the spinal chord.

-It's regular practice enhances one's digestive capabilities.

-It keeps your nervous system healthy.

-It is also found to be very helpful in healing stomach aches.

Yoga Asana #5

Vajrasan/Asana of Superlative Strength

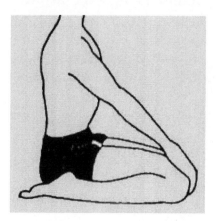

Method:

Stand straight with the waist, back and neck aligned and your feet around an inch apart.

Get down on your knees and fold your legs below your thighs.

Keep your feet spaced with the base of the feet (palms of the feet) facing upwards. (refer image)

(The nails of your fingers should touch the ground)

Easy Yoga

Then, place your bums on your heels.

Place your hands on your knees with your palms covering the knees. (keep the hands straight, don't bend them at the elbows)

All the while keep your body straight and aligned.

Be in this position for 15-20 seconds and keep breathing slowly and comfortably while you perform this Asana.

(You'll feel some discomfort in the start, so perform it for only 8-10 seconds but with regular practice you will be able to perform it for longer durations.)

Duration:

8-10 seconds when you are just starting with yoga practice, increase the duration to 7-8 minutes with regular practice.

(This is one of the few Asana's that can be performed after eating, even on a full stomach, but then reduce the duration to 3-4 minutes.)

Uses:

-This Asana helps in relieving stress and fatigue out of your legs

Advait

-People suffering from indigestion should perform this Asana after having a meal.

-It is very helpful in curing Arthritis, Back pain and other neurological disorders.

Yoga Asana #6

Vajrasan Yogamudra/Asana of Stamp in done in Vajrasan

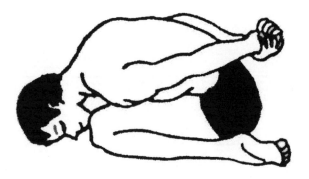

Method:

Stand straight with the waist, back and neck aligned and your feet around an inch apart.

Get down on your knees and fold your legs below your thighs.

Keep your feet spaced with the base of the feet (palms of the feet) facing upwards. (refer image)

(The surface of the nails of your toes should touch the ground)

Then, place your bums on your heels.

Place your hands on your knees with your palms covering the knees. (keep the hands straight, don't bend them at the elbows)

All the while keep your body straight and aligned. (this is the *Vajrasan* seating position)

Now bring your hands behind your back and hold the wrist of your left hand with your right hand.

Exhale and then bend forward and TRY to touch your forehead to the ground (mat).

Remain in this position for 4-5 seconds while continue breathing normally.

Then come back to your normal position.

Duration:

This Asana takes 12-15 seconds to perform and you can repeat it 3-4 times.

Uses:

-This Asana is very helpful in curing the diseases of the digestive system.

Easy Yoga

-It makes the spine, waist, back muscles and blood vessels flexible.

-It is very effective in controlling Diabetes.

-It is found to be extremely effective in Weight Loss and is very widely used to burn excess fat around the waist.

Yoga Asana #7

Sinhasan/Asana of Lion

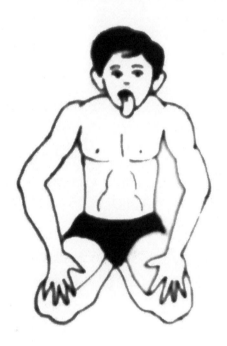

Method:

Stand straight with the waist, back and neck aligned and your feet around an inch apart.

Get down on your knees and fold your legs below your thighs.

Easy Yoga

Keep your feet spaced with the base of the feet (palms of the feet) facing upwards. (refer image)

(The surface of the nails of your toes should touch the ground)

Then, place your bums on your heels.

Place your hands on your knees with your palms covering the knees. (keep the hands straight, don't bend them at the elbows)

All the while keep your body straight and aligned. (this is the *Vajrasan* seating position)

Breathe in and then, bring out your tongue as much as you can, open your eyes wide to their fullest extent and also extend the fingers of both your hands as much as you can.

Stay in this position for 5-6 seconds, then exhale slowly and return to your normal position.

Duration:

It will take 10-13 seconds for performing this Asana and you can repeat it 2-3 times in the start and then you can slowly increase the number to 6-7 repetitions.

Uses:

Advait

-This Asana is very helpful in curing any disease related to ears, nose and throat.

-It maintains the health of your Thyroid gland.

-It is a very good exercise for your throat.

-It also maintains the health of your calf muscles and fingers.

Yoga Asana #8

Gorakshasan/Asana of Maharshi Gorakshnath

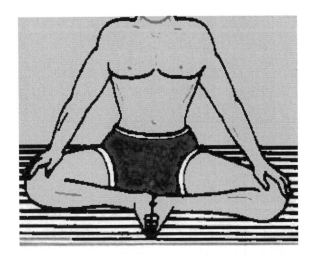

Method:

Sit comfortably on the mat with your legs stretched out front.

Now fold both your legs in such a way that the palms of your feet touch each other. (it is like doing a Namaste gesture, but with your feet.)

In this same position pull back the feet slightly so that both the heels touch the genitals.

Place both your hands on your knees and press down your knees slightly. (refer image)

Take a deep breath and hold it in and hold this position for 8-10 seconds.

Then exhale slowly and return to your normal sitting position.

Caution:

Over-Weight people and people suffering from Heart Diseases should not practice this Asana.

Duration:

It will take 15-20 seconds to perform this Asana and you can repeat it 2-3 times.

Uses:

-Regular practice of this Asana enhances fertility in men.

-It strengthens various glands in the genitals.

-It cures disorders of the urinary bladder.

-In women, this Asana is helpful in curing any menstrual disorders.

Easy Yoga

-This Asana is also used to cure pains in the waist and lower back.

Yoga Asana #9

Uttanpadasan/Asana of Leg-Lift

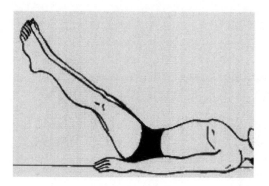

Method:

Lie down on the mat. Relax your body and bring your feet together, such that they are touching each other adjacently.

Keep your hands by your back with your palms touching the ground.

Take a deep breath, hold it in.

Now by applying pressure on the ground through your palms, raise up your legs.

Hold your legs up in the air till you can hold your breath in. (do not bend your knees, keep your legs straight.)

Then, exhale slowly and take your legs down at the same rate.

Duration:

It will take 12-15 seconds to perform this Asana and you can repeat it 2-3 times.

Uses:

-This Asana is a good detox exercise as it helps clear up the stomach.

-It strengthens the muscles of your legs and Waist.

-This Asana is very effective in burning excess fat around the stomach and the waist.

Yoga Asana #10

Shavasana / Asana of Corpse

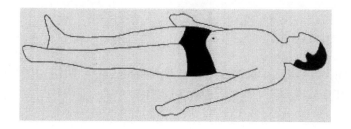

Method:

Lie down on the mat. Relax your body and bring your feet together, such that they are touching each other adjacently.

Keep your hands by your back with your palms facing upwards.

Close your eyes and breathe calmly for 10-12 seconds.

Then imagine/visualize a luminous beam of light entering your body through the top of your head and running along your spine and illuminating it.

Imagine the light entering your neck and nourishing your thyroid, and then imagine it entering your heart and bringing you more calmness.

Then imagine this light, spreading through your shoulders to your elbows and then onto your palms and then reaching and nourishing each and every finger of yours and then feel them getting relaxed completely.

Then this light overflows from your heart and fills all your chest cavity and abdomen, nourishing each and every organ in the abdomen and relaxing those organs.

Then this light, from the lower end of your spine, spreads into your hips and then flows into your legs and reaches every finger of your feet and internally nourishes them and then feel the entire lower part of your body very relaxed.

In the final phase, this light enters your face through your neck and nourishes your teeth, tongue, lips, nose, ears and eyes and then you feel those parts relaxed completely.

Keep breathing slowly and gently allow your breath to relax you more and more.

After about 10-12 minutes in this state, slowly roll to your right side while keeping your eyes closed. Stay in this state for a minute.

Then with the support of your right hand, sit up with your legs folded with eyes still closed.

Now breathe deeply, become aware of the environment around you and slowly open your eyes.

Duration:

This Asana takes around 15 minutes to perform and is to be used as a relaxation Asana.

Uses:

-It relieves you of any Stress you might have.

-It boosts internal healing.

-It works like a charm in curing hypertension.

-It is an effective cure for Insomnia.

-It is very helpful in curing Anxiety.

-It relaxes the body after a Yoga session.

How to Practice these Asana's?

The Asana's that I have mentioned are the basic exercises that will get you started with your practice of Yoga. They are to be performed for the first week or two to prepare your body for a more disciplined and extensive practice of yoga.

Start your Yoga session by practicing the 'Swastikasan' and end your session by performing the 'Shavasan'.

The remaining eight (8) Asana's are to be practiced as the core physical Asana's of the Yoga session. If you are not able to take out time to do these 8 Asana's, at a stretch, perform any four (4) of them on alternate days, but practice these Asana's regularly.

40 minutes a day is all you need and that too, for your own health.

What's Next?

This Book has laid the foundation for you to start a routine Yoga practice and the only thing that now remains, is to have a well planned set of different Asana's for each day of the week.

The upcoming book in this series is *'Monday Yoga'* and it will be released in a couple of weeks.

To receive an update when that book is released and to get amazing health & healing tips, *subscribe to my newsletter.*

Thank You!

Thank you so much for reading my book. I hope you really liked it.

As you probably know, many people look at the reviews on Amazon before they decide to purchase a book.

If you liked the book, please take a minute to leave a review with your feedback.

60 seconds is all I'm asking for, and it would mean a lot to me.

Thank You so much.

All the best,

Advait

Other Books by Advait

Mudras for Awakening Chakras: 19 Simple Hand
Gestures for Awakening & Balancing Your
Chakras

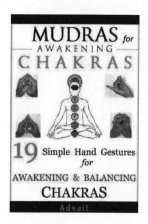

http://www.amazon.com/dp/B00P82C0AY

[#1 Bestseller in 'Yoga']

[#1 Bestseller in 'Chakras']

Easy Yoga

Mudras for Weight Loss: 21 Simple Hand
Gestures for Effortless Weight Loss

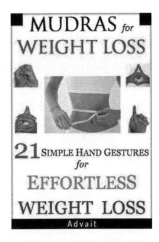

http://www.amazon.com/dp/B00P3ZPSEK

Mudras for Spiritual Healing: 21 Simple Hand
Gestures for Ultimate Spiritual Healing &
Awakening

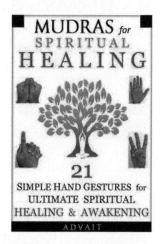

http://www.amazon.com/dp/B00PFYZLQO

Easy Yoga

Mudras for Sex: 25 Simple Hand Gestures for Extreme Erotic Pleasure & Sexual Vitality

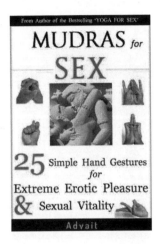

http://www.amazon.com/dp/B00OJR1DRY

Mudras: 25 Ultimate Techniques for Self Healing

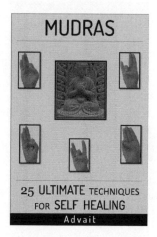

http://www.amazon.com/dp/B00MMPB5CI

Mudras of Anxiety: 25 Simple Hand Gestures for Curing Anxiety

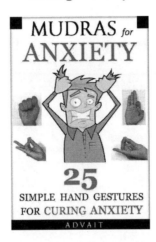

http://www.amazon.com/dp/B00PF011IU

Mudras for a Strong Heart: 21 Simple Hand
Gestures for Preventing, Curing & Reversing
Heart Disease

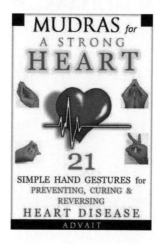

http://www.amazon.com/dp/B00PFRLGTM

Easy Yoga

Mudras for Curing Cancer: 21 Simple Hand
Gestures for Preventing & Curing Cancer

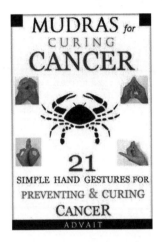

http://www.amazon.com/dp/B00PFO199M

Mudras for Stress Management: 21 Simple Hand Gestures for a Stress Free Life

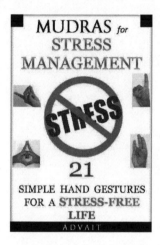

http://amazon.com/dp/B00PFTJ6OC

Easy Yoga

Mudras for Memory Improvement: 25 Simple Hand Gestures for Ultimate Memory Improvement

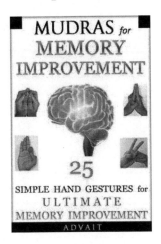

http://www.amazon.com/dp/B00PFSP8TK

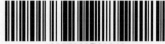

Printed in Great Britain
by Amazon.co.uk, Ltd.,
Marston Gate.